MW01536884

Date: ____________________

Time	Food	Category	Notes
Water	☐ ☐ ☐ ☐ ☐ ☐ ☐ ☐ ☐ ☐ ☐		

Date: ____________________

Time	Food	Category	Notes
Water	☐ ☐ ☐ ☐ ☐ ☐ ☐ ☐ ☐ ☐ ☐		

Date: ______________________

Time	Food	Category	Notes
Water	☐ ☐ ☐ ☐ ☐ ☐ ☐ ☐ ☐ ☐ ☐		

Date: ______________________

Time	Food	Category	Notes
Water	☐ ☐ ☐ ☐ ☐ ☐ ☐ ☐ ☐ ☐ ☐		

Date: ____________________

Time	Food	Category	Notes
Water	☐ ☐ ☐ ☐ ☐ ☐ ☐ ☐ ☐ ☐ ☐		

Date: ______________________

Time	Food	Category	Notes
Water	☐ ☐ ☐ ☐ ☐ ☐ ☐ ☐ ☐ ☐ ☐		

Date: ______________________

Time	Food	Category	Notes
Water	☐ ☐ ☐ ☐ ☐ ☐ ☐ ☐ ☐ ☐ ☐		

Date: ______________________

Time	Food	Category	Notes
Water	☐ ☐ ☐ ☐ ☐ ☐ ☐ ☐ ☐ ☐ ☐		

Date: ____________________

Time	Food	Category	Notes
Water	☐ ☐ ☐ ☐ ☐ ☐ ☐ ☐ ☐ ☐ ☐		

Date: ____________________

Time	Food	Category	Notes
Water	☐ ☐ ☐ ☐ ☐ ☐ ☐ ☐ ☐ ☐ ☐		

Date: ______________________

Time	Food	Category	Notes
Water	☐ ☐ ☐ ☐ ☐ ☐ ☐ ☐ ☐ ☐ ☐		

Date: ____________________

Time	Food	Category	Notes
Water	☐ ☐ ☐ ☐ ☐ ☐ ☐ ☐ ☐ ☐ ☐		

Date: ____________________

Time	Food	Category	Notes
Water	☐ ☐ ☐ ☐ ☐ ☐ ☐ ☐ ☐ ☐ ☐		

Date: ____________________

Time	Food	Category	Notes
Water	☐ ☐ ☐ ☐ ☐ ☐ ☐ ☐ ☐ ☐ ☐		

Date: ____________________

Time	Food	Category	Notes
Water	☐ ☐ ☐ ☐ ☐ ☐ ☐ ☐ ☐ ☐ ☐		

Date: ______________________

Time	Food	Category	Notes
Water	☐ ☐ ☐ ☐ ☐ ☐ ☐ ☐ ☐ ☐ ☐		

Date: ____________________

Time	Food	Category	Notes
Water	☐ ☐ ☐ ☐ ☐ ☐ ☐ ☐ ☐ ☐ ☐		

Date: ______________________

Time	Food	Category	Notes
Water	☐ ☐ ☐ ☐ ☐ ☐ ☐ ☐ ☐ ☐ ☐		

Date: ____________________

Time	Food	Category	Notes
Water	☐ ☐ ☐ ☐ ☐ ☐ ☐ ☐ ☐ ☐ ☐		

Date: ____________________

Time	Food	Category	Notes
Water	☐ ☐ ☐ ☐ ☐ ☐ ☐ ☐ ☐ ☐ ☐		

Date: ____________________

Time	Food	Category	Notes
Water	☐ ☐ ☐ ☐ ☐ ☐ ☐ ☐ ☐ ☐ ☐		

Date: ____________________________

Time	Food	Category	Notes
Water	☐ ☐ ☐ ☐ ☐ ☐ ☐ ☐ ☐ ☐ ☐		

Date: ____________________

Time	Food	Category	Notes
Water	☐ ☐ ☐ ☐ ☐ ☐ ☐ ☐ ☐ ☐ ☐		

Date: ____________________

Time	Food	Category	Notes
Water	☐ ☐ ☐ ☐ ☐ ☐ ☐ ☐ ☐ ☐ ☐		

Date: ____________________

Time	Food	Category	Notes
Water	☐ ☐ ☐ ☐ ☐ ☐ ☐ ☐ ☐ ☐ ☐		

Date: ____________________

Time	Food	Category	Notes
Water	☐ ☐ ☐ ☐ ☐ ☐ ☐ ☐ ☐ ☐ ☐		

Date: ____________________

Time	Food	Category	Notes
Water	☐ ☐ ☐ ☐ ☐ ☐ ☐ ☐ ☐ ☐ ☐		

Date: ____________________

Time	Food	Category	Notes
Water	☐ ☐ ☐ ☐ ☐ ☐ ☐ ☐ ☐ ☐ ☐		

Date: ______________________

Time	Food	Category	Notes
Water	☐ ☐ ☐ ☐ ☐ ☐ ☐ ☐ ☐ ☐ ☐		

Date: ______________________

Time	Food	Category	Notes
Water	☐ ☐ ☐ ☐ ☐ ☐ ☐ ☐ ☐ ☐ ☐		

Date: ______________________

Time	Food	Category	Notes
Water	☐ ☐ ☐ ☐ ☐ ☐ ☐ ☐ ☐ ☐ ☐		

Date: ____________________

Time	Food	Category	Notes
Water	☐ ☐ ☐ ☐ ☐ ☐ ☐ ☐ ☐ ☐ ☐		

Date: ____________________

Time	Food	Category	Notes
Water	☐ ☐ ☐ ☐ ☐ ☐ ☐ ☐ ☐ ☐ ☐		

Date: ____________________

Time	Food	Category	Notes
Water	☐ ☐ ☐ ☐ ☐ ☐ ☐ ☐ ☐ ☐ ☐		

Date: ______________________

Time	Food	Category	Notes
Water	☐ ☐ ☐ ☐ ☐ ☐ ☐ ☐ ☐ ☐ ☐		

Date: ______________________

Time	Food	Category	Notes
Water	☐ ☐ ☐ ☐ ☐ ☐ ☐ ☐ ☐ ☐ ☐		

Date: ___________________________

Time	Food	Category	Notes
Water	☐ ☐ ☐ ☐ ☐ ☐ ☐ ☐ ☐ ☐ ☐		

Date: ____________________

Time	Food	Category	Notes
Water	☐ ☐ ☐ ☐ ☐ ☐ ☐ ☐ ☐ ☐ ☐		

Date: ______________________

Time	Food	Category	Notes
Water	☐ ☐ ☐ ☐ ☐ ☐ ☐ ☐ ☐ ☐ ☐		

Date: ____________________

Time	Food	Category	Notes
Water	☐ ☐ ☐ ☐ ☐ ☐ ☐ ☐ ☐ ☐ ☐		

Date: ____________________________

Time	Food	Category	Notes
Water	☐ ☐ ☐ ☐ ☐ ☐ ☐ ☐ ☐ ☐ ☐		

Date: ____________________________

Time	Food	Category	Notes
Water	☐ ☐ ☐ ☐ ☐ ☐ ☐ ☐ ☐ ☐ ☐		

Date: ______________________

Time	Food	Category	Notes
Water	☐ ☐ ☐ ☐ ☐ ☐ ☐ ☐ ☐ ☐ ☐		

Date: ____________________

Time	Food	Category	Notes
Water	☐ ☐ ☐ ☐ ☐ ☐ ☐ ☐ ☐ ☐ ☐		

Date: ____________________

Time	Food	Category	Notes
Water	☐ ☐ ☐ ☐ ☐ ☐ ☐ ☐ ☐ ☐ ☐		

Date: ____________________

Time	Food	Category	Notes
Water	☐ ☐ ☐ ☐ ☐ ☐ ☐ ☐ ☐ ☐ ☐		

Date: ______________________

Time	Food	Category	Notes
Water	☐ ☐ ☐ ☐ ☐ ☐ ☐ ☐ ☐ ☐ ☐		

Date: ____________________

Time	Food	Category	Notes
Water	☐ ☐ ☐ ☐ ☐ ☐ ☐ ☐ ☐ ☐ ☐		

Date: ____________________

Time	Food	Category	Notes
Water	☐ ☐ ☐ ☐ ☐ ☐ ☐ ☐ ☐ ☐ ☐		

Date: ____________________________

Time	Food	Category	Notes
Water	☐ ☐ ☐ ☐ ☐ ☐ ☐ ☐ ☐ ☐ ☐		

Date: ______________________

Time	Food	Category	Notes
Water	☐ ☐ ☐ ☐ ☐ ☐ ☐ ☐ ☐ ☐ ☐		

Date: ____________________

Time	Food	Category	Notes
Water	☐ ☐ ☐ ☐ ☐ ☐ ☐ ☐ ☐ ☐ ☐		

Date: ______________________

Time	Food	Category	Notes
Water	☐ ☐ ☐ ☐ ☐ ☐ ☐ ☐ ☐ ☐ ☐		

Date: ______________________

Time	Food	Category	Notes
Water	☐ ☐ ☐ ☐ ☐ ☐ ☐ ☐ ☐ ☐ ☐		

Date: ______________________

Time	Food	Category	Notes
Water	☐ ☐ ☐ ☐ ☐ ☐ ☐ ☐ ☐ ☐ ☐		

Date: ____________________

Time	Food	Category	Notes
Water	☐ ☐ ☐ ☐ ☐ ☐ ☐ ☐ ☐ ☐ ☐		

Date: ____________________________

Time	Food	Category	Notes
Water	☐ ☐ ☐ ☐ ☐ ☐ ☐ ☐ ☐ ☐ ☐		

Date: ______________________

Time	Food	Category	Notes
Water	☐ ☐ ☐ ☐ ☐ ☐ ☐ ☐ ☐ ☐ ☐		

Date: ____________________

Time	Food	Category	Notes
Water	☐ ☐ ☐ ☐ ☐ ☐ ☐ ☐ ☐ ☐ ☐		

Date: ____________________

Time	Food	Category	Notes
Water	☐ ☐ ☐ ☐ ☐ ☐ ☐ ☐ ☐ ☐ ☐		

Date: ______________________

Time	Food	Category	Notes
Water	☐ ☐ ☐ ☐ ☐ ☐ ☐ ☐ ☐ ☐ ☐		

Date: ____________________

Time	Food	Category	Notes
Water	☐ ☐ ☐ ☐ ☐ ☐ ☐ ☐ ☐ ☐ ☐		

Date: ______________________

Time	Food	Category	Notes
Water	☐ ☐ ☐ ☐ ☐ ☐ ☐ ☐ ☐ ☐ ☐		

Date: ____________________

Time	Food	Category	Notes
Water	☐ ☐ ☐ ☐ ☐ ☐ ☐ ☐ ☐ ☐ ☐		

Date: ______________________

Time	Food	Category	Notes
Water	☐ ☐ ☐ ☐ ☐ ☐ ☐ ☐ ☐ ☐ ☐		

Date: ______________________

Time	Food	Category	Notes
Water	☐ ☐ ☐ ☐ ☐ ☐ ☐ ☐ ☐ ☐ ☐		

Date: ______________________

Time	Food	Category	Notes
Water	☐ ☐ ☐ ☐ ☐ ☐ ☐ ☐ ☐ ☐ ☐		

Date: ____________________

Time	Food	Category	Notes
Water	☐ ☐ ☐ ☐ ☐ ☐ ☐ ☐ ☐ ☐ ☐		

Date: ____________________

Time	Food	Category	Notes
Water	☐ ☐ ☐ ☐ ☐ ☐ ☐ ☐ ☐ ☐ ☐		

Date: ____________________

Time	Food	Category	Notes
Water	☐ ☐ ☐ ☐ ☐ ☐ ☐ ☐ ☐ ☐ ☐		

Date: ______________________

Time	Food	Category	Notes
Water	☐ ☐ ☐ ☐ ☐ ☐ ☐ ☐ ☐ ☐ ☐		

Date: ______________________

Time	Food	Category	Notes
Water	☐ ☐ ☐ ☐ ☐ ☐ ☐ ☐ ☐ ☐ ☐		

Date: ____________________

Time	Food	Category	Notes
Water	☐ ☐ ☐ ☐ ☐ ☐ ☐ ☐ ☐ ☐ ☐		

Date: ______________________

Time	Food	Category	Notes
Water	☐ ☐ ☐ ☐ ☐ ☐ ☐ ☐ ☐ ☐ ☐		

Date: ____________________________

Time	Food	Category	Notes
Water	☐ ☐ ☐ ☐ ☐ ☐ ☐ ☐ ☐ ☐ ☐		

Date: ____________________

Time	Food	Category	Notes
Water	☐ ☐ ☐ ☐ ☐ ☐ ☐ ☐ ☐ ☐ ☐		

Date: ______________________

Time	Food	Category	Notes
Water	☐ ☐ ☐ ☐ ☐ ☐ ☐ ☐ ☐ ☐ ☐		

Date: ____________________

Time	Food	Category	Notes
Water	☐ ☐ ☐ ☐ ☐ ☐ ☐ ☐ ☐ ☐ ☐		

Date: ____________________

Time	Food	Category	Notes
Water	☐ ☐ ☐ ☐ ☐ ☐ ☐ ☐ ☐ ☐ ☐		

Date: ____________________

Time	Food	Category	Notes
Water	☐ ☐ ☐ ☐ ☐ ☐ ☐ ☐ ☐ ☐ ☐		

Date: ____________________

Time	Food	Category	Notes
Water	☐ ☐ ☐ ☐ ☐ ☐ ☐ ☐ ☐ ☐ ☐		

Date: ______________________

Time	Food	Category	Notes
Water	☐ ☐ ☐ ☐ ☐ ☐ ☐ ☐ ☐ ☐ ☐		

Date: ______________________

Time	Food	Category	Notes
Water	☐ ☐ ☐ ☐ ☐ ☐ ☐ ☐ ☐ ☐ ☐		

Date: ____________________

Time	Food	Category	Notes
Water	☐ ☐ ☐ ☐ ☐ ☐ ☐ ☐ ☐ ☐ ☐		

Date: ____________________

Time	Food	Category	Notes
Water	☐ ☐ ☐ ☐ ☐ ☐ ☐ ☐ ☐ ☐ ☐		

Date: ____________________

Time	Food	Category	Notes
Water	☐ ☐ ☐ ☐ ☐ ☐ ☐ ☐ ☐ ☐ ☐		

Date: ____________________

Time	Food	Category	Notes
Water	☐ ☐ ☐ ☐ ☐ ☐ ☐ ☐ ☐ ☐ ☐		

Date: ____________________

Time	Food	Category	Notes
Water	☐ ☐ ☐ ☐ ☐ ☐ ☐ ☐ ☐ ☐ ☐		

Date: ______________________

Time	Food	Category	Notes
Water	☐ ☐ ☐ ☐ ☐ ☐ ☐ ☐ ☐ ☐ ☐		

Date: ____________________

Time	Food	Category	Notes
Water	☐ ☐ ☐ ☐ ☐ ☐ ☐ ☐ ☐ ☐ ☐		

Date: ____________________

Time	Food	Category	Notes
Water	☐ ☐ ☐ ☐ ☐ ☐ ☐ ☐ ☐ ☐ ☐		

Date: ______________________

Time	Food	Category	Notes
Water	☐ ☐ ☐ ☐ ☐ ☐ ☐ ☐ ☐ ☐ ☐		

Date: ______________________

Time	Food	Category	Notes
Water	☐ ☐ ☐ ☐ ☐ ☐ ☐ ☐ ☐ ☐ ☐		

Date: ____________________

Time	Food	Category	Notes
Water	☐ ☐ ☐ ☐ ☐ ☐ ☐ ☐ ☐ ☐ ☐		

Date: ____________________

Time	Food	Category	Notes
Water	☐ ☐ ☐ ☐ ☐ ☐ ☐ ☐ ☐ ☐ ☐		

Date: ______________________

Time	Food	Category	Notes
Water	☐ ☐ ☐ ☐ ☐ ☐ ☐ ☐ ☐ ☐ ☐		

Date: ______________________

Time	Food	Category	Notes
Water	☐ ☐ ☐ ☐ ☐ ☐ ☐ ☐ ☐ ☐ ☐		

Date: ______________________

Time	Food	Category	Notes
Water	☐ ☐ ☐ ☐ ☐ ☐ ☐ ☐ ☐ ☐ ☐		

Date: ____________________

Time	Food	Category	Notes
Water	☐ ☐ ☐ ☐ ☐ ☐ ☐ ☐ ☐ ☐ ☐		

Date: ______________________

Time	Food	Category	Notes
Water	☐ ☐ ☐ ☐ ☐ ☐ ☐ ☐ ☐ ☐ ☐		

Date: ______________________

Time	Food	Category	Notes
Water	☐ ☐ ☐ ☐ ☐ ☐ ☐ ☐ ☐ ☐ ☐		

Date: ____________________

Time	Food	Category	Notes
Water	☐ ☐ ☐ ☐ ☐ ☐ ☐ ☐ ☐ ☐ ☐		

Date: ______________________

Time	Food	Category	Notes
Water	☐ ☐ ☐ ☐ ☐ ☐ ☐ ☐ ☐ ☐ ☐		

Date: ____________________

Time	Food	Category	Notes
Water	☐ ☐ ☐ ☐ ☐ ☐ ☐ ☐ ☐ ☐ ☐		

Date: ____________________

Time	Food	Category	Notes
Water	☐ ☐ ☐ ☐ ☐ ☐ ☐ ☐ ☐ ☐ ☐		

Date: ____________________

Time	Food	Category	Notes
Water	☐ ☐ ☐ ☐ ☐ ☐ ☐ ☐ ☐ ☐ ☐		

Date: ____________________

Time	Food	Category	Notes
Water	☐ ☐ ☐ ☐ ☐ ☐ ☐ ☐ ☐ ☐ ☐		

Date: ____________________

Time	Food	Category	Notes
Water	☐ ☐ ☐ ☐ ☐ ☐ ☐ ☐ ☐ ☐ ☐		

Date: ______________________

Time	Food	Category	Notes
Water	☐ ☐ ☐ ☐ ☐ ☐ ☐ ☐ ☐ ☐ ☐		

Date: ______________________

Time	Food	Category	Notes
Water	☐ ☐ ☐ ☐ ☐ ☐ ☐ ☐ ☐ ☐ ☐		

Date: ____________________

Time	Food	Category	Notes
Water	☐ ☐ ☐ ☐ ☐ ☐ ☐ ☐ ☐ ☐ ☐		

Date: ____________________________

Time	Food	Category	Notes
Water	☐ ☐ ☐ ☐ ☐ ☐ ☐ ☐ ☐ ☐ ☐		

Date: ____________________

Time	Food	Category	Notes
Water	☐ ☐ ☐ ☐ ☐ ☐ ☐ ☐ ☐ ☐ ☐		

Date: ____________________

Time	Food	Category	Notes
Water	☐ ☐ ☐ ☐ ☐ ☐ ☐ ☐ ☐ ☐ ☐		

Date: ______________________

Time	Food	Category	Notes
Water	☐ ☐ ☐ ☐ ☐ ☐ ☐ ☐ ☐ ☐ ☐		

Date: ______________________

Time	Food	Category	Notes
Water	☐ ☐ ☐ ☐ ☐ ☐ ☐ ☐ ☐ ☐ ☐		

Date: ______________________

Time	Food	Category	Notes
Water	☐ ☐ ☐ ☐ ☐ ☐ ☐ ☐ ☐ ☐ ☐		

Date: ____________________

Time	Food	Category	Notes
Water	☐ ☐ ☐ ☐ ☐ ☐ ☐ ☐ ☐ ☐ ☐		

Date: ____________________

Time	Food	Category	Notes
Water	☐ ☐ ☐ ☐ ☐ ☐ ☐ ☐ ☐ ☐ ☐		

Date: ______________________

Time	Food	Category	Notes
Water	☐ ☐ ☐ ☐ ☐ ☐ ☐ ☐ ☐ ☐ ☐		

Date: ______________________

Time	Food	Category	Notes
Water	☐ ☐ ☐ ☐ ☐ ☐ ☐ ☐ ☐ ☐ ☐		

Date: ______________________

Time	Food	Category	Notes
Water	☐ ☐ ☐ ☐ ☐ ☐ ☐ ☐ ☐ ☐ ☐		

Date: ____________________

Time	Food	Category	Notes
Water	☐ ☐ ☐ ☐ ☐ ☐ ☐ ☐ ☐ ☐ ☐		

Date: ______________________

Time	Food	Category	Notes
Water	☐ ☐ ☐ ☐ ☐ ☐ ☐ ☐ ☐ ☐ ☐		

Date: ____________________

Time	Food	Category	Notes
Water	☐ ☐ ☐ ☐ ☐ ☐ ☐ ☐ ☐ ☐ ☐		

Date: ____________________

Time	Food	Category	Notes
Water	☐ ☐ ☐ ☐ ☐ ☐ ☐ ☐ ☐ ☐ ☐		

Date: ____________________

Time	Food	Category	Notes
Water	☐ ☐ ☐ ☐ ☐ ☐ ☐ ☐ ☐ ☐ ☐		

Date: ____________________

Time	Food	Category	Notes
Water	☐ ☐ ☐ ☐ ☐ ☐ ☐ ☐ ☐ ☐ ☐		

Date: ____________________

Time	Food	Category	Notes
Water	☐ ☐ ☐ ☐ ☐ ☐ ☐ ☐ ☐ ☐ ☐		

Date: ______________________

Time	Food	Category	Notes
Water	☐ ☐ ☐ ☐ ☐ ☐ ☐ ☐ ☐ ☐ ☐		

Date: ______________________

Time	Food	Category	Notes
Water	☐ ☐ ☐ ☐ ☐ ☐ ☐ ☐ ☐ ☐ ☐		

Date: ____________________

Time	Food	Category	Notes
Water	☐ ☐ ☐ ☐ ☐ ☐ ☐ ☐ ☐ ☐ ☐		

Date: ____________________

Time	Food	Category	Notes
Water	☐ ☐ ☐ ☐ ☐ ☐ ☐ ☐ ☐ ☐ ☐		

Date: ______________________

Time	Food	Category	Notes
Water	☐ ☐ ☐ ☐ ☐ ☐ ☐ ☐ ☐ ☐ ☐		

Date: ____________________

Time	Food	Category	Notes
Water	☐ ☐ ☐ ☐ ☐ ☐ ☐ ☐ ☐ ☐ ☐		

Date: ____________________

Time	Food	Category	Notes
Water	☐ ☐ ☐ ☐ ☐ ☐ ☐ ☐ ☐ ☐ ☐		

Date: ____________________

Time	Food	Category	Notes
Water	☐ ☐ ☐ ☐ ☐ ☐ ☐ ☐ ☐ ☐ ☐		

Date: ______________________

Time	Food	Category	Notes
Water	☐ ☐ ☐ ☐ ☐ ☐ ☐ ☐ ☐ ☐ ☐		

Date: ____________________

Time	Food	Category	Notes
Water	☐ ☐ ☐ ☐ ☐ ☐ ☐ ☐ ☐ ☐ ☐		

Date: ____________________

Time	Food	Category	Notes

Water	☐	☐	☐	☐	☐	☐	☐	☐	☐	☐	☐

Date: ____________________

Time	Food	Category	Notes
Water	☐ ☐ ☐ ☐ ☐ ☐ ☐ ☐ ☐ ☐ ☐		

Date: ____________________

Time	Food	Category	Notes
Water	☐ ☐ ☐ ☐ ☐ ☐ ☐ ☐ ☐ ☐ ☐		

Date: ______________________

Time	Food	Category	Notes
Water	☐ ☐ ☐ ☐ ☐ ☐ ☐ ☐ ☐ ☐ ☐		

Date: ____________________

Time	Food	Category	Notes
Water	☐ ☐ ☐ ☐ ☐ ☐ ☐ ☐ ☐ ☐ ☐		

Date: ____________________

Time	Food	Category	Notes
Water	☐ ☐ ☐ ☐ ☐ ☐ ☐ ☐ ☐ ☐ ☐		

Date: ____________________

Time	Food	Category	Notes
Water	☐ ☐ ☐ ☐ ☐ ☐ ☐ ☐ ☐ ☐ ☐		

Date: ____________________

Time	Food	Category	Notes
Water	☐ ☐ ☐ ☐ ☐ ☐ ☐ ☐ ☐ ☐ ☐		

Date: ______________________

Time	Food	Category	Notes
Water	☐ ☐ ☐ ☐ ☐ ☐ ☐ ☐ ☐ ☐ ☐		

Date: ______________________

Time	Food	Category	Notes
Water	☐ ☐ ☐ ☐ ☐ ☐ ☐ ☐ ☐ ☐ ☐		

Date: ______________________

Time	Food	Category	Notes
Water	☐ ☐ ☐ ☐ ☐ ☐ ☐ ☐ ☐ ☐ ☐		

Date: ______________________

Time	Food	Category	Notes
Water	☐ ☐ ☐ ☐ ☐ ☐ ☐ ☐ ☐ ☐ ☐		

Date: ______________________

Time	Food	Category	Notes
Water	☐ ☐ ☐ ☐ ☐ ☐ ☐ ☐ ☐ ☐ ☐		

Date: ______________________

Time	Food	Category	Notes
Water	☐ ☐ ☐ ☐ ☐ ☐ ☐ ☐ ☐ ☐ ☐		

Date: ______________________

Time	Food	Category	Notes
Water	☐ ☐ ☐ ☐ ☐ ☐ ☐ ☐ ☐ ☐ ☐		

Date: ______________________

Time	Food	Category	Notes
Water	☐ ☐ ☐ ☐ ☐ ☐ ☐ ☐ ☐ ☐ ☐		

Date: ____________________

Time	Food	Category	Notes
Water	☐ ☐ ☐ ☐ ☐ ☐ ☐ ☐ ☐ ☐ ☐		

Date: ____________________

Time	Food	Category	Notes
Water	☐ ☐ ☐ ☐ ☐ ☐ ☐ ☐ ☐ ☐ ☐		

Date: ______________________

Time	Food	Category	Notes
Water	☐ ☐ ☐ ☐ ☐ ☐ ☐ ☐ ☐ ☐ ☐		

Date: ____________________

Time	Food	Category	Notes
Water	☐ ☐ ☐ ☐ ☐ ☐ ☐ ☐ ☐ ☐ ☐		

Date: ____________________

Time	Food	Category	Notes
Water	☐ ☐ ☐ ☐ ☐ ☐ ☐ ☐ ☐ ☐ ☐		

Date: ______________________

Time	Food	Category	Notes
Water	☐ ☐ ☐ ☐ ☐ ☐ ☐ ☐ ☐ ☐ ☐		

Date: ____________________

Time	Food	Category	Notes
Water	☐ ☐ ☐ ☐ ☐ ☐ ☐ ☐ ☐ ☐ ☐		

Date: ____________________

Time	Food	Category	Notes
Water	☐ ☐ ☐ ☐ ☐ ☐ ☐ ☐ ☐ ☐ ☐		

Date: ____________________

Time	Food	Category	Notes

Water	☐	☐	☐	☐	☐	☐	☐	☐	☐	☐	☐

Date: ______________________

Time	Food	Category	Notes
Water	☐ ☐ ☐ ☐ ☐ ☐ ☐ ☐ ☐ ☐ ☐		

Date: ____________________

Time	Food	Category	Notes
Water	☐ ☐ ☐ ☐ ☐ ☐ ☐ ☐ ☐ ☐ ☐		

Date: ______________________

Time	Food	Category	Notes
Water	☐ ☐ ☐ ☐ ☐ ☐ ☐ ☐ ☐ ☐ ☐		

Date: ______________________

Time	Food	Category	Notes
Water	☐ ☐ ☐ ☐ ☐ ☐ ☐ ☐ ☐ ☐ ☐		

Date: ______________________

Time	Food	Category	Notes
Water	☐ ☐ ☐ ☐ ☐ ☐ ☐ ☐ ☐ ☐ ☐		

Date: ____________________

Time	Food	Category	Notes
Water	☐ ☐ ☐ ☐ ☐ ☐ ☐ ☐ ☐ ☐ ☐		

Date: ____________________

Time	Food	Category	Notes
Water	☐ ☐ ☐ ☐ ☐ ☐ ☐ ☐ ☐ ☐ ☐		

Date: ____________________

Time	Food	Category	Notes
Water	☐ ☐ ☐ ☐ ☐ ☐ ☐ ☐ ☐ ☐ ☐		

Date: ____________________

Time	Food	Category	Notes
Water	☐ ☐ ☐ ☐ ☐ ☐ ☐ ☐ ☐ ☐ ☐		

Date: ______________________

Time	Food	Category	Notes
Water	☐ ☐ ☐ ☐ ☐ ☐ ☐ ☐ ☐ ☐ ☐		

Date: ____________________

Time	Food	Category	Notes
Water	☐ ☐ ☐ ☐ ☐ ☐ ☐ ☐ ☐ ☐ ☐		

Date: ____________________

Time	Food	Category	Notes
Water	☐ ☐ ☐ ☐ ☐ ☐ ☐ ☐ ☐ ☐ ☐		

Date: ____________________

Time	Food	Category	Notes
Water	☐ ☐ ☐ ☐ ☐ ☐ ☐ ☐ ☐ ☐ ☐		

Date: ______________________

Time	Food	Category	Notes
Water	☐ ☐ ☐ ☐ ☐ ☐ ☐ ☐ ☐ ☐ ☐		

Date: ____________________

Time	Food	Category	Notes
Water	☐ ☐ ☐ ☐ ☐ ☐ ☐ ☐ ☐ ☐ ☐		

Date: ______________________

Time	Food	Category	Notes
Water	☐ ☐ ☐ ☐ ☐ ☐ ☐ ☐ ☐ ☐ ☐		

Date: ____________________

Time	Food	Category	Notes
Water	☐ ☐ ☐ ☐ ☐ ☐ ☐ ☐ ☐ ☐ ☐		

Date: ____________________

Time	Food	Category	Notes
Water	☐ ☐ ☐ ☐ ☐ ☐ ☐ ☐ ☐ ☐ ☐		

Date: ______________________

Time	Food	Category	Notes
Water	☐ ☐ ☐ ☐ ☐ ☐ ☐ ☐ ☐ ☐ ☐		

Date: ______________________

Time	Food	Category	Notes
Water	☐ ☐ ☐ ☐ ☐ ☐ ☐ ☐ ☐ ☐ ☐		

Date: ______________________________

Time	Food	Category	Notes
Water	☐ ☐ ☐ ☐ ☐ ☐ ☐ ☐ ☐ ☐ ☐		

Date: ____________________

Time	Food	Category	Notes
Water	☐ ☐ ☐ ☐ ☐ ☐ ☐ ☐ ☐ ☐ ☐		

Date: ______________________

Time	Food	Category	Notes
Water	☐ ☐ ☐ ☐ ☐ ☐ ☐ ☐ ☐ ☐ ☐		

Date: ____________________

Time	Food	Category	Notes
Water	☐ ☐ ☐ ☐ ☐ ☐ ☐ ☐ ☐ ☐ ☐		

Date: ____________________

Time	Food	Category	Notes
Water	☐ ☐ ☐ ☐ ☐ ☐ ☐ ☐ ☐ ☐ ☐		

Date: ____________________

Time	Food	Category	Notes
Water	☐ ☐ ☐ ☐ ☐ ☐ ☐ ☐ ☐ ☐ ☐		

Date: ____________________

Time	Food	Category	Notes
Water	☐ ☐ ☐ ☐ ☐ ☐ ☐ ☐ ☐ ☐ ☐		

Date: ______________________

Time	Food	Category	Notes
Water	☐ ☐ ☐ ☐ ☐ ☐ ☐ ☐ ☐ ☐ ☐		

Date: ____________________

Time	Food	Category	Notes
Water	☐ ☐ ☐ ☐ ☐ ☐ ☐ ☐ ☐ ☐ ☐		

Date: ______________________

Time	Food	Category	Notes
Water	☐ ☐ ☐ ☐ ☐ ☐ ☐ ☐ ☐ ☐ ☐		

Date: ______________________

Time	Food	Category	Notes
Water	☐ ☐ ☐ ☐ ☐ ☐ ☐ ☐ ☐ ☐ ☐		

Date: ______________________

Time	Food	Category	Notes
Water	☐ ☐ ☐ ☐ ☐ ☐ ☐ ☐ ☐ ☐ ☐		

Date: ____________________________

Time	Food	Category	Notes
Water	☐ ☐ ☐ ☐ ☐ ☐ ☐ ☐ ☐ ☐ ☐		

Date: ____________________

Time	Food	Category	Notes
Water	☐ ☐ ☐ ☐ ☐ ☐ ☐ ☐ ☐ ☐ ☐		

Date: ______________________

Time	Food	Category	Notes
Water	☐ ☐ ☐ ☐ ☐ ☐ ☐ ☐ ☐ ☐ ☐		

Date: ____________________

Time	Food	Category	Notes
Water	☐ ☐ ☐ ☐ ☐ ☐ ☐ ☐ ☐ ☐ ☐		

Made in the USA
Coppell, TX
03 June 2022

78425416R00111